Prentice Hall's Exploring Biology Series

ALZHEIMER'S DISEASE

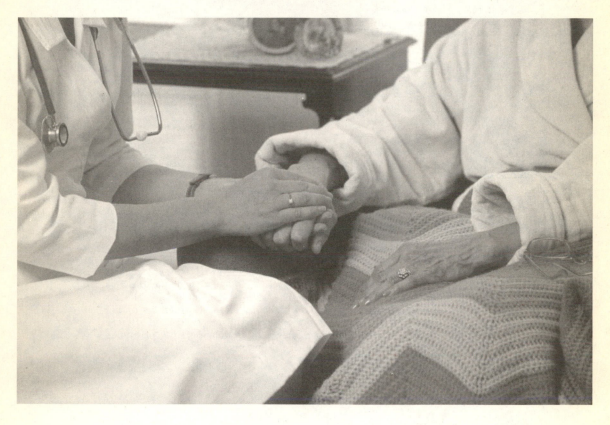

ROGER KNOWLES

DREW UNIVERSITY

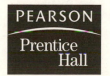

PEARSON

Prentice
Hall

Pearson Prentice Hall
Upper Saddle River, NJ 07458

Editor-in-Chief, Life and Geosciences: Sheri L. Snavely
Executive Editor: Gary Carlson
Project Manager: Crissy Dudonis
Vice President of Production & Manufacturing: David W. Riccardi
Executive Managing Editor: Kathleen Schiaparelli
Assistant Managing Editor: Becca Richter
Production Editor: Dana Dunn
Supplement Cover Management/Design: Paul Gourhan
Manufacturing Buyer: Ilene Kahn
Assistant Formatting Manager: Bill Johnson
Art Editor: Adam Velthaus
Cover Photograph: Ron Chapple/Getty Images

© 2004 Pearson Education, Inc.
Pearson Prentice Hall
Pearson Education, Inc.
Upper Saddle River, NJ 07458

The author and publisher of this book have used their best efforts in preparing this book. These efforts include the development, research, and testing of the theories and programs to determine their effectiveness. The author and publisher make no warranty of any kind, expressed or implied, with regard to these programs or the documentation contained in this book. The author and publisher shall not be liable in any event for incidental or consequential damages in connection with, or arising out of, the furnishing, performance, or use of these programs.

Printed in the United States of America

10 9 8 7 6 5 4 3 2 1

ISBN 0-13-183834-2

Pearson Education Ltd., *London*
Pearson Education Australia Pty. Ltd., *Sydney*
Pearson Education Singapore, Pte. Ltd.
Pearson Education North Asia Ltd., *Hong Kong*
Pearson Education Canada, Inc., *Toronto*
Pearson Educación de Mexico, S.A. de C.V.
Pearson Education—Japan, *Tokyo*
Pearson Education Malaysia, Pte. Ltd.
Pearson Education, *Upper Saddle River, New Jersey*

To George and Sandy

Table of Contents

Preface   *vii*

The Face of Alzheimer's Disease   *1*
    Aging, senility, and dementia   1
    Progression of dementia in AD   2
    The cost of AD   3

What's Going Wrong in AD: The Pathology   *4*
    Dementia and the degeneration of neuronal networks   4
    The search for a killer   4
    Suspect 1: Plaques   6
    Suspect 2: Tangles   10
    Suspect 3: Conspirators   12

The Role of Genes in Developing AD   *13*
    Familial versus sporadic AD   13
    Genetics and early-onset AD   14
    Inheriting mutations in three genes can lead to Early-onset AD   15
    A possible common pathway for the genes responsible for Early-onset AD   15
    APOE and Late-onset AD   17
    Genes and the risk of AD   19

The Role of the Environment in Developing AD   *20*
    The immune System: Too much of a good thing?   20
    Does failure to stimulate the brain lead to AD?   21
    Other environmental influences   26

Current and Future Strategies for Treating AD   *27*
    Preventing or removing plaques   28
    Protecting neurons   29

Summary   *30*

References and Suggested Readings   *30*

Preface

To say that the study of Alzheimer's disease (AD) is one of the greatest challenges facing scientists and physicians today is to believe the impact of this horrible disease. With over 4 million Americans currently diagnosed with AD, and with scientists warning us that tens of millions of people around the world will develop the disease over the coming decades, one realizes that this is a problem of global proportions. The fear of developing AD, a condition in which one slowly loses the most precious of possessions, one's memories, personality and sense of self, haunts nearly all who have come in contact with an AD patient. The disease extends beyond the patient to the patient's family and how they are devastated by seeing a parent reduced to incoherence or a spouse who no longer recognizes his or her beloved.

In the face of such personal loss, it seems churlish to even consider the economics of the disease, but as a society the financial burden of having to take care of a burgeoning demented population demands attention. Current estimates are in the $100 billion range for the annual cost of AD to the US economy. With an expected increase in the numbers of AD patients and the hope for some effective, albeit expensive, treatments, the financial burden of AD to today's young adults will be enormous.

Because of the vast scope of how AD will affect all of our lives, from personal, to social, to economic, it is imperative that a broad range of individuals understand the fundamentals about this complex disease. This book is written with the goal of informing a diverse group of students about AD as well as individuals who have been touched by the specter of AD. All will find some of the answers to questions that we have about this devastating disease.

The story of AD is an evolving one as tens of thousands of researchers work every day to expand our knowledge of the genesis of this disease and what leads to its inexorable progression. New and potentially exciting strategies for developing effective treatments are constantly being tested in laboratories. Rarely does a month go by without a report on AD in the popular press. Because of this, one important goal of this booklet is to provide the reader with the necessary skills to interpret findings from new studies and to put in context commentary that is provided to the public. When I first started doing experimental research into AD in the early 1990's at Harvard University, a well-respected scientist was quoted by the press as saying that because of his latest findings, an effective treatment for AD should be available within five years. At the time, I imagined my career as an AD researcher would be as short lived as that of a polio researcher who started right before Jonas Salk announced the discovery of an effective polio vaccine. However, my mentor at the time, a neurologist at Harvard Medical School, pointed out that his own career had already spanned several "a cure will be ready in five years" cycles and that focusing on the predictions of scientists was less productive than trying to understand how their current findings fit in with our understanding of AD.

In this book, we will start with the most vital component of any disease: the impact of the disease on the patient. After describing how the mental processes of an AD patient are affected, we will explore what is physically going wrong inside of an AD patient's brain with an emphasis placed on how the physical changes alter the way a patient can think. Then we will discuss some current theories on why people develop AD by looking at the roles of genetics and environment. Finally, we will explain how some of the current treatments for AD work and discuss a few of the possible directions for new treatment strategies.

The Face of Alzheimer's Disease

Sarah could not say when the decline began. Years after Frank had been diagnosed with probable Alzheimer's disease (AD), Sarah thought back about her husband's behavior when he was in his 60's and wondered how much of it was just Frank being Frank and how much of it was the beginning stages of a disease that would slowly rob the man she loved for the last 45 years of his memories and his ability to think clearly. For years Sarah had been getting more and more frustrated with how Frank had been acting. She thought he had been "conveniently forgetting" to do his chores or pull his share of duties at the office where they ran their small family business. She viewed it as a flaw in his character that he was not excited about travel, even to visit their adult children and grandchildren who were living in various locations across the country. Whenever she did convince him to go, he would almost immediately after arrival begin to pester her about when they should go back home. The stories were the worst. Frank would tell her something trivial, like the neighbors had been over that morning to ask them to pick up their newspaper for the next few days, and then Frank would tell Sarah again and again throughout the afternoon about the neighbors and how they should pick up their newspaper. It was as if, Sarah had thought, Frank didn't think that she could remember even the simplest of instructions.

In hindsight, after Frank's physician had given her the news about her husband's illness, Sarah realized the irony of her emotions. Frank had been repeating those stories because his brain could not recall that he had already told them to her. Sarah learned from Frank's physician that one of the qualities of AD was the insidious nature of its onset. As opposed to a stroke, where it is often easy to mark the start of the damage to the brain and the corresponding changes in one's behavior due to that damage, in AD the alterations in the brain start slowly with subtle differences in behavior that often go unnoticed. The changes also mimic some of the alterations in behavior that society expects to occur during the aging process. For example, Frank was no longer productive at the office, but then he was over the age of 65, an age when society expects people to want to retire. Frank frequently forgot to do things, yet we have grown up thinking that the medical language that describes the aging process (senility) means that a person is forgetful.

AGING, SENILITY, AND DEMENTIA

It is common to hear someone, particularly an older person, say, "I must be getting senile," upon forgetting a conversation, a person's name, or the location of one's keys. The common use of the word implies aging with memory loss. Medically, however, senile simply refers to being of a certain age. No particular deficit is implied.

Yet the association between memory loss and aging is a strong one. One reason might be the prevalence among the elderly of diseases of the brain that affect one's memory. In 2000, there were 35 million Americans aged 65 or older. Over 5 million of them suffered from diseases that robbed them of their memories. Of those, 4 million Americans had AD. 360,000 new cases are diagnosed every year. The single biggest risk factor for developing AD is age. Starting at the age of 65, the probability of developing AD doubles every five years. Of the 4 million Americans who are 85 years or older, around 40% have AD. The following table shows the percentage of Americans in different age groups who have AD.

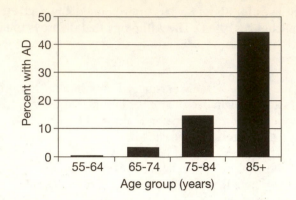

Dementia was coined as a medical term in the early 1800's to refer to people who had a disruption in their mental processes. In modern times, clinicians define dementia as a condition that severely impairs both short and long term memory as well as at least one other mental process (judgment, abstract thinking, language, recognition, personality, etc.) to such an extent that these disturbances interfere with daily living. There are many diseases that can lead to dementia, including Prion diseases (one of which is "Mad Cow Disease"), Lewy body disease, Huntington disease, and Alzheimer's disease. Each disease has a different presentation of dementia. For example, in Huntington disease, patients lose control of their motor skills such that their limbs will jerk uncontrollably. In Prion diseases, the onset of dementia is abrupt and the progression of mental loss is very rapid.

PROGRESSION OF DEMENTIA IN AD

In AD, the onset and progression of dementia is slow and gradual. In the case of Frank, his wife noticed changes in his behavior for nearly 7 years before he was diagnosed with AD. Four years later, Frank still recognized his wife, but had trouble recognizing his own children. Frank went from reading four to six non-fiction books a month before he was diagnosed with AD, to starting and then forgetting to finish reading a dozen books a year, to re-reading the same passage from the same book over and over, to finally enjoying just holding a book, any book, open on his lap and looking at the pages without making any sense of the words or ideas contained within. During the early stages, Sarah could invite long time friends over to dinner and know that while Frank might not be able to follow the conversation, he would occasionally interject with a story (which he would repeat several times throughout the evening), and he would get comfort from their company. As the disease progressed, Frank became more and more anxious during social situations, often making rude remarks or pestering his wife to make people leave. Four years after his diagnosis, Frank routinely sat mutely when friends visited, not even trying to follow conversations. If Sarah tried to leave a room without him, he would follow her, not wanting to be left alone for a minute. He wouldn't even let her vacuum in the next room without coming to hover around her. If Frank follows the typical progression of dementia of AD, over the next 4 years he will continue to lose language and reasoning skills to the point where he will be mostly mute, and when he does communicate, the majority of it will be nonsense. Frank has lived in the same house for over 40 years, yet within a year or two; he will have trouble recognizing his surroundings and could easily get hopelessly lost in the town that he's lived in most of his life.

Typically an AD patient lives for about 8 years after being diagnosed. However, death is not due directly to the physical changes of AD. The pathology that destroys the brain is not directly lethal. If the body otherwise remains healthy, and caregivers continue to feed and nourish the patient, an AD patient can live for decades with this horrible disease. When a patient is said to have died of AD, the cause of death is usually from a secondary condition like pneumonia or sepsis from infection.

THE COST OF AD

The burden of AD on individuals like Frank and his wife Sarah are immeasurable. For Frank, the act of slowly sinking into a mental fog that never lifts, but just gets murkier, is horrifying. Besides progressive dementia, two of the most common symptoms of AD are clinical depression and anxiety. At least half of all patients need to take anti-depressants or anti-anxiety medication. At the beginning of his disease, Frank was self-aware enough to realize that it was getting harder and harder to think. Later, that self-awareness was replaced by a childlike fear of the unknown. Unfortunately, with his memory shot and so little left that seemed familiar, even the act of his wife stepping out of the room for just a moment left him terrified. Sarah's suffering was different, but just as dramatic. The stress and burden of caring for her husband was and is physically and emotionally exhausting. She can't leave him alone and is forced to watch after him even on mundane excursions to the supermarket. Conversation is painful as Frank repeatedly asks the same question over and over, never remembering that Sarah just a moment ago gave him the answer. Her biggest joy in life is visiting her nine grandchildren, yet Frank is even harder to keep calm when they travel. Finally, she fears that her own memory of Frank as a caring, vibrant, and intelligent man will forever be replaced with the face of Alzheimer's disease.

While the costs to patients and their families are incalculable, the economic cost of AD is not. In a 2002 report prepared by the Alzheimer's Association, the cost to American businesses was estimated at $61 billion annually. This figure included the loss in productivity of caregivers like Sarah as well as the business share of health care costs to patients. Since most people do not have insurance to cover long term care, families of AD patients often have to pay out of pocket for nursing home care (which nationally averages $42,000 per year). Combined with the impact on business, the total costs of AD run upward of $100 billion a year.

The economic future looks bleaker. The over-85-year-old segment of the population is the fastest growing, meaning that the number of patients is going to skyrocket. Some estimates suggest that 14 million Americans will have AD by 2050. If medical research on AD does not make rapid progress, the number of Americans working full time to care for a large demented population will be vast. Even if the bio-medical community successfully develops effective treatment or preventative strategies for AD by the middle of the 21st century, one can presume that the price of treatment will not be inexpensive and that has implications for the quality of life of those supporting AD patients.

What's Going Wrong in AD: The Pathology

DEMENTIA AND THE DEGENERATION OF NEURONAL NETWORKS

A year and a half after Frank had been diagnosed with AD, he had a conversation with his son-in-law on one of his favorite subjects, World War II. Frank described how WWII was one of the central events of his life. Even though his son-in-law was clearly in his thirties, having been born some 20 years after the end of WWII, Frank asked him whether he had fought in the war. Two years later, during a conversation with his son-in-law, Frank could not recall which countries the US fought during WWII. In this example, Frank's deteriorating mental faculties can clearly be seen. At first, memories, such as the life altering events of WWII, could be recalled. However, by asking whether his son-in-law had fought in WWII, Frank demonstrated he had clear deficits taking that memory and using it appropriately in conversation. Two years later, the memory itself deteriorated to the point where he was unable to recall who had been fighting in the war.

The ability to recall memories is due to a physical process that occurs in the brain. This process is based upon neurons that communicate with each other by the processing of electrical signals from one side of a neuron to another, and by the release of chemicals from one neuron to the next neuron. The neurons are arranged in complex networks that are responsible for discrete functions within the brain. To use a memory in conversation, such as knowing whether it is appropriate to ask a man in his 30's if he fought in a war that ended over 50 years ago, additional neural networks need to be employed. The pattern of neurons communicating with each other that encodes the memory of the war must be sent to a large set of neurons involved in a working memory. Once there, the part of the memory that has encoded Frank's age is compared to Frank's perception of the age of his son-in-law. This perception of age is also encoded by neurons communicating with each other. The physical space in the brain where Frank's judgment exists also results from sets of neurons communicating with each other. In other words, the act of going from just recalling a memory to the act of using that memory in productive behavior requires an exponential increase in the total amount of messages that need to be sent from one set of neurons to another.

Given this understanding of how the biology of the mind works, the simplest explanation of what is going wrong with Frank's brain is that the ability of large sets of neurons to communicate with each other is gradually degrading. Early in the disease, Frank was able to accurately recall a memory using a neuronal network that appeared to be functionally intact; however, he was unable to manipulate the memory in his brain to generate appropriate conversation, a task requiring neural networks to "talk" to each other. Later in the disease state, Frank was unable to describe important details of his memory of WWII, probably because the neurons that were involved in encoding that memory could no longer communicate with each other effectively.

THE SEARCH FOR A KILLER

What could have created this deterioration in Frank's neurons' ability to communicate with each other? From as early as 1907, when Alois Alzheimer first characterized the physical changes that occurred in the brain of a demented woman, many scientists have focused on plaques and tangles as the most likely culprits. Plaques and tangles are the distinguishing pathological lesions in the brains of AD patients, which mean that a patient is not given a "definitive" diagnosis of AD until both plaques and tangles are detected in the patient's brain. Because it is impossible with today's technology to see plaques and tangles inside a living patient's brain, this definitive diagnosis, unfortunately, is not possible until the patient dies. Using imaging devices like Magnetic Resonance Imaging (MRI) and Positron Emission Tomography (PET), however, doctors can look inside a living patient's brain and detect regions of the brain that are smaller or using less energy, both signs that neuronal networks are being destroyed.

To distinguish whether plaques and tangles are a consequence of the disease or a driving force for the progression of AD, researchers carefully examined the brains of AD patients after they died. This allowed them to study one particular time in a patient's life in some detail. They got to observe how many plaques and tangles there were throughout the brain and where they were located (Figure 1). They were able to test whether the chemical or molecular nature of different structures

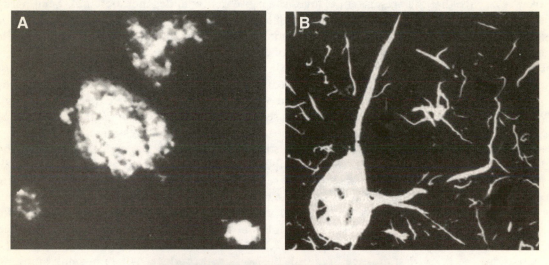

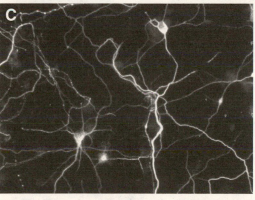

Figure 1
A. Extracellular deposits of A-beta form plaques in the brain of a patient who had AD. **B**. Tangle inside of a neuron from a patient who had AD. The neuron's soma is the white pear shaped structure in the lower left, with the curly cue lines representing tangles in the neuron's axons and dendrites. **C**. Pictures of normal healthy neurons grown in cell culture. The long lines are the axons and dendrites making connections with each other.

within the brain were different compared to the brain of someone who had died without having AD. What scientists could not and cannot do is test whether there is causality involved. They cannot watch as a plaque destroys neurons or tangles break apart a neuronal network, because those are processes that only occur while the patient is alive. Therefore, these types of studies are similar to that of a crime investigator arriving at the scene of a murder and looking for evidence of who did the killing. But as opposed to most murder mysteries where the evidence is scant and the suspects have fled the scene, in AD, there are many suspects hanging around and nearly all of them are acting as if they are guilty.

SUSPECT #1: PLAQUES

At this time, the vast majority of research into AD is focused on figuring out how plaques form in the brain of AD patients and what can be done to stop this formation. Partly this is due to the strong evidence that the presence of plaques can cause neuronal degeneration in AD, but partly it is also due to the relative accessibility of plaques as compared to the other things that might be going wrong in AD. Unlike tangles which form inside of neurons, and thus may be hard to reach, let alone fix, plaques form around the outside of neurons in the spaces between cells in the brain. This means that if plaques are responsible for breaking up neuronal networks and thus the loss of a patient's ability to think clearly, then researchers need only figure out a way to break the plaques apart or clear them out in some way, in order to develop an effective treatment strategy. We will discuss possible treatment strategies in section 5. Here we will examine the evidence that plaques are at least partially responsible for the development and progression of AD.

First, what are plaques? Basically they are sticky, gunky, circular deposits that form around neurons. Just like trying to understand the plaques that stick to the walls of your blood vessels and that can lead to vascular disease, brain researchers have spent much time trying to figure out what the substances are that make up neuronal plaques and where this material comes from. The major component of plaques is a molecule called "amyloid-beta" or A-beta for short. A-beta is a small molecule, one of several that come from a much larger protein called "amyloid precursor protein" (APP) (Figure 2). Interestingly, APP is a protein that is found throughout the body, and most cell types in the body will produce A-beta in small amounts. But researchers only find A-beta plaques in the brain, suggesting that there is something specific about the brain environment that leads to the formation of A-beta plaques. All of the plaques found in AD have A-beta as one of their components. Because of this, scientists view A-beta as an essential component of the plaques, and thus a likely suspect in the case of the deteriorating neuronal networks.

Figure 2
The A-beta fragment is generated by cutting the full length Amyloid Precursor Protein (APP) at the location of the two arrows. This A-beta fragment is either digested inside of the cell, or released into the spaces between cells.

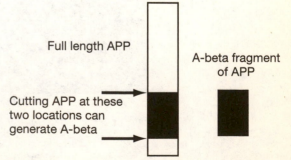

In order to figure out what is going on, scientists first like to propose a hypothesis, an educated guess, such as "The formation of A-beta into plaques causes neuronal networks to deteriorate in AD patients." From that hypothesis, scientists can then make a series of predictions that would follow *if* the hypothesis were true. They then design an experiment to see if the predictions were correct and whether the results could be replicated by other scientists. If the predictions are not matched by experimental results, scientists go back to the drawing board to come up with alternative hypotheses. Here are three predictions from the above hypothesis:

Prediction #1: A-beta will form into plaque-like structures in a test tube.

Prediction #2: A-beta will cause degeneration of neurons in culture.

Prediction #3: Generating A-beta plaques in an animal will lead to AD-like behavior.

When scientists conducted the experiments to test these predictions, they generally found evidence to support the overall hypothesis. There were some interesting caveats, however. In the experiments to test prediction #1 (A-beta will form into plaque-like structures in a test tube.), A-beta only formed aggregates that had plaque-like characteristics when the concentration of the A-beta was very high or when the solution became very acidic. From this, researchers wondered whether something in the brain of AD patients was causing A-beta to accumulate in specific locations, and that as more of it accumulated, the concentration of it went up, leading to the formation of plaques. If this were the case, maybe it is not the A-beta itself which is the problem, but whatever is acting as a magnet to attract it to a variety of spots in the brain. It is also intriguing that the degree of acid build up increases A-beta forming plaque-like structures. Increase in the production of molecules called "free radicals" can lead to increased acidity, and the elderly are more prone to build up of these free radicals. This suggests to some that this might be the reason for AD being primarily a disease of the elderly.

When scientists conducted research into prediction #2 (A-beta will cause degeneration of neurons in culture.), whether A-beta can destroy neurons in culture (through a method whereby scientists take neurons harvested from the brains of rats or mice), the early results were mixed. In some experiments, it looked like A-beta was a deadly toxin – killing 80% of the neurons over a two-day period. In other experiments, A-beta acted as a growth factor promoting the survival of neurons. As researchers tried to resolve these diametrically opposed results, two important factors became apparent. The first was that if the A-beta was allowed to aggregate like it does in plaques, then A-beta becomes more toxic. This made sense because if A-beta is normally produced by all cells (including neurons), then coming in contact with A-beta under relatively normal circumstances shouldn't be deadly to the neurons. Only with the aggregation found in plaques would one expect A-beta to be harmful to neurons. The second factor that influenced whether A-beta was toxic or not was the number of amino acids in the molecule. Amino acids are simply the building blocks for proteins whose sequence (the order in which they are put together) are determined by the strand of DNA that encodes for a particular gene. In this case, there is a gene that codes for APP and it produces a protein that can be anywhere from 670 to 717 amino acids long. It turns out that when APP is cut into smaller fragments, several different sizes of A-beta are made. Around 90% of the A-beta that is produced is 40 amino acids long and about 10% is 42 amino acids long. The A-beta that is 42 amino acids long appears to be the more toxic of the two. This has led some to propose the idea that one of the events that might be going wrong in AD is a shift to a higher ratio of A-beta that is 42 amino acids long. In the next section we will look at the case of a gene that when mutated in several places may lead to this increase in the longer form of A-beta.

The research into prediction #3 (Generating A-beta plaques in an animal will lead to AD-like behavior.) has been fairly controversial. A genetically engineered strain of mice produces A-beta plaques. The number of plaques in the brains of these experimental mice is significantly greater than that found in AD patients, yet the level of behavior changes is not great and the loss and degeneration of neurons has been minor. The lack of drastic changes in behavior can partly be attributed to the sophistication of the animal. For example, earlier we looked at the case of Frank who after having AD for about 18 months could tell a good WWII story, though he clearly had trouble applying that knowledge in conversation. Most of the studies with mice have tested their ability to learn things like a simple radial arm maze or poking their nose at a lever after having plaques in their brains for 1-2 years. These tasks may require relatively simple neuronal networks to operate effectively. If that is true, modest degeneration of neurons may not lead to easily detected behavioral changes. And while there has not been a huge loss of neurons in these mice, that is not surprising given that neuronal loss is a gradual process in AD.

There are some interesting twists in considering A-beta as the prime suspect in the case of the deteriorating neuronal networks. First, when one looks at the brains of individuals who have AD, one finds that there is no link between the amount of plaques in the brain and the length of time that an individual had AD. In other words, if someone were in the beginning stages of AD, such that the ability to think coherently were reduced, but not the ability to recognize the faces of family members, that person could have the same number of A-beta plaques as an individual who had the disease for over a decade and no longer recognized a spouse. The lack of correlation between the duration of the disease, the cognitive effects of the disease, and the presence of these plaques does not fit well with the general idea that A-beta plaques are the prime neuronal killers in AD. To go along with this, plaques in low numbers can be found in the brains of the elderly who do not exhibit any of the mental declines that are associated with AD at the time of their death. Finally, in AD, plaques will often form in parts of the brain that function normally. For example, plaques may form in a part of the visual system even though vision does not decline in AD. These puzzling observations suggest to researchers that while A-beta may be *essential* to the formation of the plaques, the presence of A-beta is not *sufficient* to turn the plaques into destructive agents.

There is plenty of evidence, however, to suggest that something bad is happening around at least a subset of the plaques. Instead of looking at just the presence of A-beta, scientists have examined the physical structure of neurons in and around the plaques' locations and have indeed found that at the very least, a subset of plaques can mark the location where much damage is done (Figure 3). Some researchers are trying to find out if various cells and molecules that associate with plaques can combine with A-beta and result in neuronal degeneration. Examples of these include heavy metals, an abnormal accumulation of molecules involved in clearing fat or cholesterol, immune cells that may be "accidentally" destroying neurons, and molecular signals that may be telling the neurons to "commit suicide." The idea here is that one or more of these other events must occur in order to turn a rather benign plaque into one that systematically destroys the neurons in and around it.

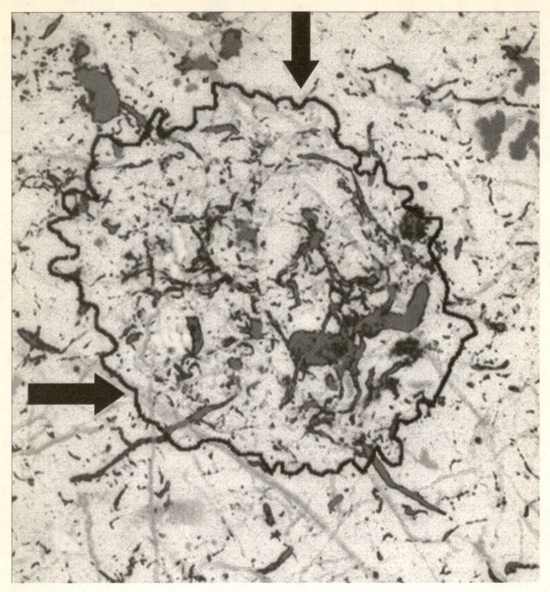

Figure 3
A picture taken of a brain section from an AD patient. The arrows point to the outline of the location of a plaque. The dark squiggly lines are tangle bearing axons and dendrites from affected neurons. Notice that there is a higher degree of tangles inside of the plaque than in the area outside of the plaque.

SUSPECT #2: TANGLES

As opposed to plaques, tangles are a physical change that occurs *inside* neurons during the course of the disease. Another important difference between plaques and tangles is that when a tangle forms inside of a neuron, it is always damaging and leaves the neuron twisted and deformed, and unable to function as efficiently as before.

Why is the shape of a neuron so important? Part of the reason a neuron is able to receive information from many other neurons and then send that information to many distant neurons is that it is able to maintain a unique and functional form. The contour of a neuron is determined both genetically and by experiences which mold the specific connective parts of the neuron—called synapses—that link one neuron to another. For example, your genes help determine that the neurons whose function it is to recognize faces have long connective projections called axons that connect to your language centers. It is your personal experiences, however, that fine tune the shape of the axon such that neurons which respond when they recognize the face of your Aunt May have axons that specifically connect to neurons in your language center that encode for the name, "Aunt May." If the shape of these axons changes slightly, they may instead connect to the neurons that encode for the name "Uncle Ben," which could prove to be embarrassing, to say the least.

In AD, tangles cause the neuron to lose the integrity of its shape, thereby disrupting the intricately connected neurons that communicate with each other to produce meaningful mental activity. That in itself would be enough to make tangles a likely suspect in what's causing deterioration in neuronal networks, but to make the case even more compelling, there is a tighter correlation between the appearance of tangles and deficits in mental ability than there is with plaques and cognitive decline. The number of tangles found in an AD patient's brain is directly related to the length of time the person had the disease at the time of death. In other words, an individual who had the disease for just a year before passing away would have fewer tangles than someone who had the disease for three years before dying, and that person would have fewer tangles than someone who had AD for 5 years, and so on. Additionally, the location of tangles in the brain would match very closely with behavioral deficits. For example, an AD patient who had no problems with control of motor functions but who had trouble speaking in sentences would have no tangles present in motor areas of the brain but would have many tangles in language areas.

Interestingly, elderly people who do not have any clinical symptoms of AD often have scattered tangles in a part of the brain called the hippocampus. The hippocampus is involved in processing memory from a very short-term storage area in the brain (lasting there for just seconds) to a longer storage area (which can last minutes, hours, days, lifetimes). Imagine that you drive to the mall to watch a movie, and the movie is a big blockbuster so that by the time you arrive, the lot where you normally park is full so you have to drive around to another part of the mall to park. You watch the movie and when you come out, you look for your car. If your hippocampus is working well, you will go straight to the other side of the mall where you parked your car. If your hippocampus is a bit overloaded, you will go to your usual lot first before remembering where you parked the car. If your hippocampus is not functioning at all, you would go to your usual lot and then either call the police or search randomly through the parking lot until you found it (and pray that you are not in the Mall of America). Going back to the elderly, it is a common complaint of older adults that they have trouble remembering things that depend upon the hippocampus, like where they parked the car or the details of a recent conversation. A biological reason to explain this complaint is the appearance of tangles in the hippocampus as one ages.

As in the research into plaques, scientists have spent great effort trying to figure out what exactly tangles are and how they are produced. Given that tangles cause neurons to become malformed, it is not surprising that the molecule that is most highly altered in tangles is one that is involved in generating and maintaining a neuron's shape. The molecule in question is called Tau and one of its normal functions in neurons is to keep the neuron's internal skeleton, called the cytoskeleton, firm and stable. If the Tau molecule malfunctions, the cytoskeleton in parts of the neuron is likely to fall apart, resulting in the misshapen contours of a tangle-bearing neuron. To make matters worse, the Tau inside the tangle-bearing neuron changes chemically such that it forms tough fibers called "paired helical filaments." Usually when something unwanted builds up inside of neurons, there are tiny garbage disposals that can degrade the junk. Paired helical filaments, however, are so strong they can't be broken apart by the neuron's garbage disposal and so they just fill up space inside of the neuron, making it even harder for the neuron to function normally.

In general, less is known about how tangles are made than how plaques are made. The major chemical difference between Tau in a tangle versus Tau in a normal neuron is that a lot of phosphate groups get added to the Tau in tangles. Unlike Tau in normal neurons, the many additional phosphate groups attached to Tau in neuronal tangles sticks around for a long time (Figure 4). Because of this, scientists have hypothesized that changing how these phosphate groups are added to Tau will lead to the appearance of tangles and the destruction of neuronal networks in AD. Two predictions from this hypothesis have been tested:

Prediction #1: Attaching many phosphate groups to Tau will lead a neuron to develop an abnormal shape.

Prediction #2: Attaching phosphate groups to Tau will lead to the formation of paired helical filaments.

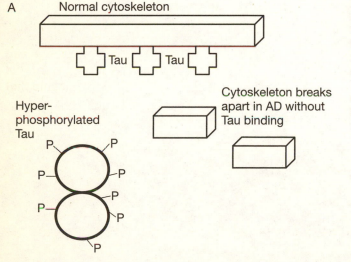

A

Normal cytoskeleton

Tau   Tau

Hyper-phosphorylated Tau

P   P
P   P
        P
P   P
    P

Cytoskeleton breaks apart in AD without Tau binding

Figure 4
In a normal brain, Tau (represented as crosses) binds to the cytoskeleton creating long stable bundles to help maintain the neuron's shape. In AD, Tau becomes hyper-phosphorylated and changes its shape to look like a "figure 8." When it is in this shape, it cannot bind to the cytoskeleton, and the bundles break apart and the neuron gets a "tangled" appearance.

Scientists have demonstrated in experiments in neuronal cell culture that excessively attaching phosphate groups to Tau causes Tau to detach from the cytoskeleton. This in turn causes the axon in the neuron to have a curved and twisted shape. The change in shape reduces the neuron's ability to communicate effectively with other neurons in its network. While this work supporting prediction #1 is promising, scientists have not yet been able to get Tau to form into the paired helical filaments that are found in AD by attaching phosphate groups to it. Thus, prediction #2 still lacks experimental support. Additional research will determine whether other chemical changes to Tau that may be going on in AD patients' neurons are responsible for forming the nearly indestructible fibers that clog up tangle bearing neurons.

SUSPECT #3: CONSPIRATORS

Scientists usually have a bias when trying to figure out why an individual develops a disease and that is: we like to look for a single cause. From a mother nagging her child, "Come in from out of the rain, or you'll catch a cold," to advertising campaigns warning us that smoking causes cancer, our society is inundated with the imagery of a single cause for a disease. In some cases, and for some diseases, that view is appropriate. For example, individuals can develop AIDS because they share a needle with a drug user who has HIV infection. However, in AD, there may be no one reason why the disease develops and progresses, but rather a convergence of several different factors that interact with each other, each participating in the slow march of doom that is the hallmark of the disease. Instead of the neuron killer being either plaques or tangles, it could be a combination of both interacting with each other to slowly tear apart the intricate tapestry of the brain. In the next two sections, we will explore other factors such as the inherited form of a particular gene (section 3) or exposure to certain environmental influences (section 4) that drive the production and lethal progression of plaques and tangles.

The Role of Genes in Developing AD

Frank's mother developed AD when she was in her late 60's. Frank was diagnosed with AD at the age of 68. When Frank's four adult children heard the news, the first thing they worried about was the health and well being of their father. That worry was quickly followed by the deep concern over how their mother would handle the stress of living and caring for her husband who was progressively losing his mind, while at the same time maintaining her home and running a small family-owned business. Each of Frank's four children, now in their 30's with families of their own, admitted that underneath their deep love and empathy for their parents, bubbled a personal and deep-seated fear. Lurking undetected in the depths of their brains, was there a ticking genetic time bomb waiting to go off, waiting to strike and rob them of their memories? When they held up their children, Frank's grandchildren, they wondered if besides passing on traits like hair color and the shape of a nose, had they also passed along a defective gene that destined them to a similar horrible fate?

FAMILIAL VERSUS SPORADIC AD

In the previous section we discussed how scientists examined the pathologies of AD as a way of trying to understand what is causing the disease and eventually how to treat it. Another powerful tool researchers use to look for causes of a disease is the study of epidemiology. Epidemiology is the study of figuring out what factors or characteristics make a person at risk for developing a particular disease. These factors can be either environmental or genetic.

To explore a potential genetic cause for AD, researchers first looked to see if AD ran in families. By sampling a population of AD patients, they found that somewhere between 25–40% of AD patients had a close family relative (sibling, parent, grandparent, aunt or uncle) who also had AD. These AD patients, like Frank, are considered to have "familial AD" while those who did not have a family member afflicted with AD are considered to have "sporadic AD."

This distinction between familial and sporadic AD does not by itself demonstrate a genetic versus environmental cause for developing the disease. Consider the case of Linda, a woman in her late 80's who was the only person in her family who had been diagnosed with AD, and thus would be considered to have sporadic AD. A closer examination of her family history, however, shows that only one of her close relatives lived past the age of 65 (and that individual was an uncle considered fairly eccentric in his later years, and thus may have had undiagnosed AD). Linda may well have a gene that carries an increased risk of AD, but her parents and grandparents, who may have developed the disease if they lived long enough, died before any symptoms might have appeared. Moreover, in the case of Frank, just because his mother also had AD, does not necessarily mean that a gene is responsible for his developing the disease. Growing up, he lived with his mother for 18 years, and during that time, both of them could have been exposed to an environmental toxin that led to the pathologies of AD.

GENETICS AND EARLY-ONSET AD

There have been a number of large families where the magnitude of affected relatives is huge. In these families, the children of a parent who has AD have a 50% chance of developing the disease. This is considered very strong evidence that in these families, AD is being caused by the inheritance of a mutation in a single gene. The biology of understanding this type of inheritance is fairly straightforward. Each person has two sets of 23 chromosomes – one set inherited from the mother, the other from the father. Each set of 23 chromosomes encodes for exactly the same type of genes so that each person has exactly two copies of each gene (the only exception is that males inherit an "X" chromosome from their mothers and a "Y" chromosome from their fathers, and thus have only one copy of each parent's genes on these "sex" chromosomes). While two copies of a particular gene will produce basically the same protein (the gene product), there may at times be slight differences between the instructions of these two genes that may in turn lead to a slightly different chemical composition of the resultant proteins. The different chemical composition of these proteins may work together to create a characteristic that is the melding of the two. Or, as in the case of these families afflicted with AD, the trait comes from just one of the two variations of proteins.

Families that carry one of the variations of the genes that can lead directly to developing AD are hit doubly hard. First, the probability of inheriting the bad copy of the gene from an affected parent is 1 in 2 (Figure 5). Second, as opposed to the other cases of AD, where the average age of onset is in the late 60's to early 70's, those that have the autosomal dominant inherited form can develop AD as early as their late 30's to as late as their mid 50's. Clinicians refer to these individuals as having early-onset AD. The cause of their developing the disease is clearly distinct from the majority who develop the disease later. Those who develop AD later are often referred to as having late-onset AD. The early-onset form of AD (which is less than 10% of the total cases of AD) is thought to accelerate more rapidly, but that might simply reflect society's expectations of a person's mental capability at different times in a person's life. If someone is no longer actively engaged in work or community, any decline in the ability of the brain to process information is frequently judged to be less dramatic than for an individual who is younger and expected to be heavily occupied in work or community activities.

Interestingly, the first case of dementia that was presented by the German physician Alois Alzheimer in 1906 which described the pathologies of plaques and tangles was a patient named Auguste D. She had been diagnosed with dementia when she was 51 years old and had died five years later. In Alzheimer's presentation, he referred to her as having presenile dementia because

Figure 5

A pedigree chart of an extended family which carries an autosomal dominant inherited trait. An affected man married an unaffected woman (top row). They had 3 children. Two of their children inherited the trait from their father (middle row). Each of the 3 children married and had children of their own. The child from the second generation that did not have the trait is at no risk of passing the trait down to her children (far right). The two affected children in the second generation pass down the trait to some of their children (bottom row).

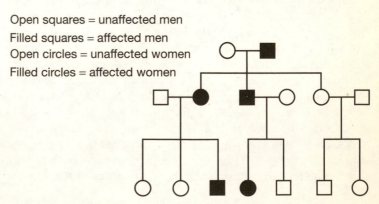

Open squares = unaffected men
Filled squares = affected men
Open circles = unaffected women
Filled circles = affected women

she was so young when she started to lose her mental faculties. By 1910, the medical profession started referring to patients who developed dementia by their 50's as having Alzheimer's disease. Those patients who developed dementia after the age of 60 were labeled as having senile dementia and were not considered to have typical AD. For decades this distinction was being made, fueled partly because family members and physicians rarely asked for a detailed autopsy of an elderly person who had suffered a dramatic mental decline. Because of this, only the rarer, Early-onset form of AD was being heavily investigated. Finally, in the 1960's reports finally came out linking most cases of senile dementia as the late-onset form of AD.

INHERITING MUTATIONS IN THREE GENES CAN LEAD TO EARLY-ONSET AD

Three genes have been identified that lead directly to inheriting early-onset AD. These three genes encode for Amyloid Precursor Protein (APP), Presenilins-1 (PS-1), and Presenilins-2 (PS-2). Mutations in specific locations of the DNA code for these three genes lead to the generation of APP, PS-1 and PS-2 proteins that have a slight change in the composition of their amino acids. This small alteration in amino acids can lead the proteins to cause development of plaques and tangles in the brain at a relatively young age.

Why do these genes cause AD in afflicted families? Scientists have spent the last few years trying to understand how these genes and the proteins that they make work inside of the brain to better get a sense of what is going wrong. As of 2002, over 70 specific mutations in the molecular code of these genes have been identified with early-onset AD. One approach to understanding the problem has been to introduce these genes with and without the particular AD changes to experimental animals and then to observe what happens. In most cases, the AD forms of the genes either generate plaques in the brains of the genetically altered animals or make it easier for the plaques to form. This is strong evidence that in the case of early-onset AD, the disease is generated from molecules in the brain making plaques. In contrast, these mutated genes do not cause the formation of tangles or cause massive loss of neurons in the experimental animal models.

A POSSIBLE COMMON PATHWAY FOR THE GENES RESPONSIBLE FOR EARLY-ONSET AD

How do these AD variants of the proteins APP, PS-1 and PS-2 work to generate plaques in patient's brains? Researchers have been asking this question from the time these genes were discovered, not just to understand what is happening in the families that have these genetic variants, but also to learn more about how plaques can be made. If these plaques cause the specific physical change in the brain that leads to disruption of neuronal networks and the horrible progression of the disease, then knowing more about how they are formed may prove very useful in creating effective medical treatments for AD.

In section 2, we discussed how the major component of plaques is a small molecule called A-beta, which is made from the larger protein APP. Since the gene for APP is one of those where specific mutations can lead to early-onset AD, then it seems reasonable to suspect that specific mutation sites are involved in plaque formation. In fact, although the protein APP can consist of as many as 717 amino acids, changes in only 7 of them can lead to early-onset AD. All 7 sites are located around the parts of APP that are cleaved to form A-beta. The consequences of these changes around the cleavage sites are such that patients who have these mutations are either producing more A-beta or are producing more of the A-beta that is 42 amino acids long. This change in amino acid length is important because as we discussed in the previous section, when A-beta is 42 amino acids long, it is more deadly to neurons than when it is just 40 amino acids long.

By 1991, scientists had discovered the gene for APP and its relationship to early-onset AD. As they considered the significance of the mutations that produce either more total A-beta or more A-beta 42, they proposed three mechanisms that might be important. First, there is a molecule called alpha-secretase which cuts APP in the middle of the A-beta sequence, and thereby prevents the formation of A-beta. Second, there is a molecule called beta-secretase which cuts APP at one end of the A-beta sequence, and thereby produces more total A-beta. Finally, there is a third molecule called gamma-secretase which cuts APP at the other end of the A-beta sequence and as it does so, produces either a 40 or a 42 amino acid long molecule. At the time, researchers did not know which molecules were the alpha, beta or gamma secretases (Figure 6).

About five years later, the genes for PS-1 and PS-2 were discovered and mutations were identified that led to early-onset AD (these molecules were called presenilins because mutations in them lead to AD prior to reaching the age of senility). At that time, many scientists thought that this would mean that another mechanism might be important for generating plaques. Then it was discovered that the mutations in the presenilins led to production of more A-beta 42. In order to test whether the presenilins are part of the gamma secretase which is responsible for producing A-beta 42, researchers inhibited PS-1 and PS-2 inside of cells. The results from these experiments were fairly conclusive: gamma secretase activity decreased by 80%. Researchers have now conducted molecular experiments that have provided strong evidence that the presenilins are part of the complex of molecules that make up the gamma secretase. In other words, the presenilins are involved in cutting APP at the site where more of the toxic A-beta 42 can be formed. This suggests that rather than discovering a new pathway inside of cells that can generate plaques, the discovery of the presenilins have confirmed that the cleavage of APP into various sized fragments is a crucial element in the genesis of early-onset AD. While there are no mutations in the genes encoding APP, PS-1 and PS-2 in the more common late-onset AD, there may be environmental or age-related events that cause these molecules to act differently within cells, thereby generating destructive plaques.

Figure 6
Location where the 3 secretases cut APP. Alpha-secretase cuts APP in the middle of the A-beta fragment, preventing A-beta from forming. Beta-secretase cuts at one end of the A-beta fragment, and gamma-secretase at the other end. Gamma-secretase can cut either 40 or 42 amino acids away from where Beta-secretase cuts, causing A-beta to be either the short or the long form. The 42 amino acid form of A-beta is thought to be the more toxic of the two.

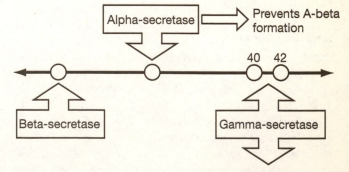

APOE AND LATE-ONSET AD

The mutations in APP, PS-1 and PS-2 are rare within the general population and only account for a small segment of those affected with AD. In the case of Frank, because he was not diagnosed with AD until he was 68, he in all likelihood does not carry one of the genetic variants for APP, PS-1 or PS-2. However, that does not necessarily mean that he does not carry a form of a gene that influenced his development of AD, and if passed down to his children, increases their risk for developing this terrible disease. In the mid-1990's, researchers found a fairly common form of a gene called APOE which was associated with a large number of late-onset AD patients. There are three common forms of APOE, called E2, E3, and E4 and in the general population, about 30% of people have at least one copy of the E4 type. If one looked at just those with late-onset AD, about 50% have at least one copy of the E4 type. Examining just the cases of late-onset AD where there is a family history of AD (like Frank and his mother), 75% of those have at least one copy of the E4 type of the APOE gene.

So that means that Frank has a 3 out of 4 chance of having an E4 type of APOE gene. If he does, and only has one copy of the E4 (with the other copy being an E2 or an E3), then each of his children would have a 50% chance of inheriting an E4 type from him. If Frank has two copies of the E4 type, then each of his children would inherit an E4 from him. Does that mean that either half or all of Frank's children will develop AD? The answer is no. As opposed to the early-onset AD cases where everyone who inherits the "bad" forms of APP, PS-1 or PS-2 will eventually develop AD, with APOE, the AD trait is not solely determined by the inheritance of a gene type. A good number of individuals have lived to be quite old and never developed AD while carrying an E4 APOE gene type. Likewise, even though half of AD patients have the E4 type, half do not. The scientific conclusion is that rather than considering the inheritance of a type of APOE as a cause for AD, researchers consider it to be a risk factor for AD.

Less is known about the mechanism of how the E4 form of APOE can influence the development of the AD. As opposed to APP, PS-1, and PS-2, APOE does not have an obvious role in producing A-beta. Rather than having a function inside of neurons, the APOE gene is produced by support cells in the brain called glial cells, and then secreted into the spaces between the cells. Evidence suggests that APOE normally works by doing two things: delivering needed resources to neurons and getting rid of junk that accumulates outside of the cells. Scientists have speculated that one or both of these functions is being disrupted in AD, and that the E4 form of APOE is more likely to have a loss of function than the other two forms (E2 and E3).

One of the resources that APOE can deliver to neurons is lipids (a type of molecule that does not dissolve in water, like fats). Among other applications, neurons use lipids to maintain their outer coating, called the plasma membrane. Lack of sufficient lipids for neurons can lead to a loss of synapses connecting neurons together, and thus a decrease in the ability of neurons to communicate with each other in the intricate pattern that generates mental activity. In AD, the plaques that form around neurons have a lot of APOE binding to them. Some scientists have suggested that when APOE binds to the plaques, it is unable to do its normal job of delivering lipids to neurons, and thus makes the neurons more susceptible to the damage that the plaques are doing to them. If this is the case, then perhaps the E4 form of APOE gets stuck to the plaques more easily than the other forms, making individuals with E4 more likely to have damage to their neuronal networks (Figure 7). This hypothesis proposes that inheriting one form of APOE versus another does not impact whether plaques will develop, but rather how much damage the plaques might do.

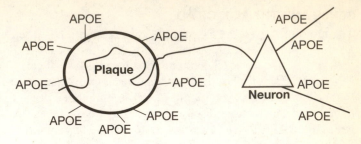

Figure 7

Neurons can take up APOE, giving the axons and dendrites the lipids (fat molecules) to keep them healthy. Plaques can attract and bind APOE, preventing the APOE in that area from being delivered to neurons. This may cause the axons and dendrites that pass through the plaque to appear curved and not as good at communicating with other neurons.

Another hypothesis implies that APOE can influence generation of AD pathologies. One thing that has puzzled researchers is why plaques form in the first place when there are robust clearance mechanisms in the brain, such as microglia, which specialize in getting rid of unwanted substances in the spaces between neurons. What's more, these microglial cells often surround the plaques in the brains of AD patients. One way that A-beta gets cleared in the brain is that it binds to APOE and the resultant A-beta/APOE complex is taken up by microglia. Some experiments suggest that the E4 form of APOE does not bind as well as the other forms of APOE, making it harder to get rid of the A-beta, and allowing it to accumulate to form plaques (Figure 8). This hypothesis implies that APOE affects the generation of plaques not from the inside of neurons like APP, PS-1 and PS-2, but rather from outside of neurons.

There are two major implications that can be drawn from each of these hypotheses on how APOE can influence the development of AD. First, by itself, the inheritance of one form of APOE is not sufficient to generate AD in a patient. Both proposed mechanisms require something to happen within the brain to cause the neurons to begin to produce a large quantity of A-beta before the E4 form of APOE begins to contribute to the formation of the pathologies of AD. Second, both mechanisms point to possible strategies for combating the physical changes that occur due to the pathogenesis of AD. If neurons are being damaged partly due to a failure of receiving enough lipids, maybe growth factors can be used to stimulate lipid production and overcome this deficit. If plaques are forming in part due to the inability of APOE to get rid of the A-beta, maybe another clearance mechanism can be stimulated to help microglia get rid of this unwanted molecule.

Figure 8

Microglia cells act as scavengers, getting rid of unwanted junk around neurons. When the E2 or E3 form of APOE binds to A-beta, it may form a shape that easily fits into a receptor on the microglia, allowing the APOE/A-beta complex to be easily digested. When the E4 form of APOE binds to A-beta, it may form a shape that is not as easily taken up by the microglia.

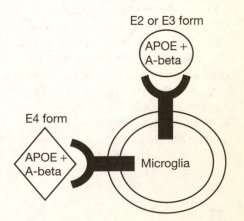

GENES AND THE RISK OF AD

About half of the cases of early-onset AD are caused by the defects in APP, PS-1 or PS-2. Scientists are hopeful that with the information provided by the human genome project, the genetic causes for the other half of the early-onset AD cases can be identified. For the more common late-onset form of AD, the only conclusive genetic risk factor that has been identified so far has been the inheritance of the E4 form of APOE. Inheritance of the E4 form of APOE is only considered a risk factor, and not a cause, because it increases the probability of developing AD, but by itself does not cause the disease. Several other genetic risk factors have been suggested recently, but none of these candidate genes have been conclusively tested in a large population.

Gene	Type of AD	Risk factor or Cause	% of Total AD cases
APP	Early-onset	Cause	<1 %
PS-1	Early-onset	Cause	3–5%
PS-2	Early-onset	Cause	1%
Unknown	Early-onset	Unknown	3–5%
APOE	Late-onset	Risk factor	50%
Unknown	Late-onset	Unknown	40%

The Role of the Environment in Developing AD

With the exception of the small segment of AD patients who carry the mutant forms of APP, PS-1 and PS-2 which lead to early-onset AD, scientists are fairly certain that the environment plays a role in who and when a person develops AD. How much of a role is unclear. Many feel that a convergence and accumulation of factors, both genetic and environmental, lead to the onset of the physical changes that bring about AD. However, it is not inconsequential to examine the role the environment plays in the development of diseases in a population. No two people ever experience the same environmental factors. Children born in the same family within a few years of each other will have very distinct interactions with their surroundings, generating different phenotypes based upon the order in which siblings were born.

Researchers often define environment as anything that mediates a person's interactions with the physical world. From the clothes you wear to the food you eat, from movies you watch to conversations you have, from the air you breathe to the time you sleep, all represent environmental factors. Some even define environment as any factor other than genes that influences a body's functions. For example, cardiovascular disease can be due to either a genetic pre-disposition or the way one treated one's body (too many french fries, too little exercise) or some combination. A personal history of cardiovascular disease can in turn be a non-genetic factor that influences whether a person develops another disease. In this case, it would not matter whether someone had a heart attack because of the influence of genes or McDonalds, but rather the consequences of such things as decreased blood flow, decreased oxygen consumption, and weakening of blood vessels.

When looking at diseases of the brain, like AD, it is important to consider the range of things that can influence the structure and function of the components of the nervous system. These factors can include things like head trauma, drug use, and exposure to toxins. Environmental factors that influence the brain can also include things that modulate how we engage in mental activities. We will look at two factors, response of the immune system and education.

THE IMMUNE SYSTEM: TOO MUCH OF A GOOD THING?

In simplistic terms a body's immune system is its defense against illness and injury. Specialized cells and anatomical areas respond to things like infections, cuts, and contusions by producing a response designed to limit the damage and to rid the body of the agents causing the problems. The immune system does this in two ways, by making the environment inhospitable to foreign invaders by doing things like raising the temperature of the body and by directing immune cells to the site of infection to actively fight whatever does not belong in the host body.

However, this explanation implies that there is some over-arching director overseeing the body's response, and this is not the case. Each immune cell is programmed to make its decisions about what to do based upon what it senses in its environment. These cells have molecules called receptors which enable them to pick up signals about what is happening around them and then respond. Sometimes these immune cells are tricked into thinking a signal is coming from an outside intruder when in fact the signal is coming from the host's own body. The immune cells will then attack parts of its own body, causing some serious damage. This is called auto-immune disease. Physicians treat auto-immune patients by giving them drugs which suppress the person's immune cells from attacking anything. These patients are considered immune-compromised because their body will not act robustly to attack an infection and they thus require a lot of follow-up care by their physicians to make sure that normally mild common illnesses do not lead to severe complications.

Interestingly, doctors began to notice that these immune-compromised patients rarely had AD, even as they aged into their 70's and 80's. A study was conducted that demonstrated that individuals who took medication that suppressed their immune system were less likely to develop AD. Even common over-the-counter medication like ibuprofen was effective in reducing the risk of developing AD.

Why would weakening the immune system help prevent AD, unless some of the immune cells were somehow contributing to the pathologies of AD? That was the question a number of researchers have posed recently, and a likely suspect are the microglial cells in the brain. In section 3, we discussed that microglial cells were in and around plaques and that they had a role in trying to get rid of the A-beta that was forming into clumps. Microglial cells are also immune cells, and one hypothesis is that their receptors are "viewing" the plaques as a foreign substance to attack, and thus are releasing chemicals called cytokines (which are proteins that act to mobilize other immune cells to aggressively attack the site of infection) and a gas called nitric oxide to try to defeat the plaques (Figure 9). However, as they are doing that, they may also inadvertently be damaging the neurons that are around the plaques, contributing to the degeneration of neuronal communication seen in AD. If this hypothesis is supported by further research, it would mean that individuals who take immune suppressing medication may have plaques develop, but those plaques will not cause as much damage to the neurons around them as they do in AD.

DOES FAILURE TO STIMULATE THE BRAIN LEAD TO AD?

For nearly two hundred years neuroscientists have proposed the idea that the brain is like a muscle in that the more one uses it, the stronger it gets. In 1807, Franz Joseph Gall, a physician who studied the anatomy of the brain suggested that discrete areas of the brain got bigger when a person used that part of the brain for mental activities. Ramon y Cajal, considered by many to be the father of modern neurobiology, proposed in the early 1900's that the connections between the neurons, the synapses, would increase in number and get stronger with repeated use. Over the last couple of decades, researchers have provided strong experimental evidence that indeed the cortex of the brain (the area of the brain that houses all of the neuronal cell bodies and most of the synapses) can change in thickness due to environmental stimulation. Prolonged inactivity can lead to a decrease in thickness and a loss of number of synapses, while high level of mental activity can lead to an increase in thickness and a gain in number of synapses.

In AD, one of the consequences of the pathologies of plaques and tangles is that there is a loss of synapses and a decrease in thickness of cortex in areas of the brain that correlate to the specific mental declines seen in patients. Areas related to learning and memory are hit hard early in the disease, followed by centers involved in emotion, language, recognition, and judgment. In addition, AD patients brains' use less energy, even when they are asked to perform simple mental tasks that they can successfully complete. This is fairly strong evidence that as one prominent neuroscientist described it, AD is a condition of "synaptic failure" (Selkoe, 2002).

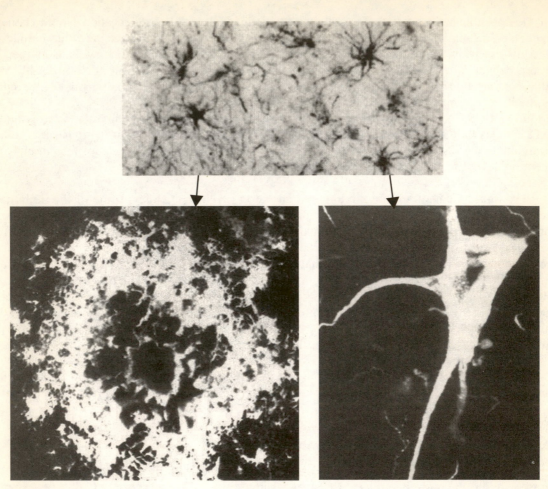

Figure 9
Microglia (top) can be activated by plaques (bottom left) to release gases and chemicals which can damage invaders. Unfortunately, neurons (bottom right) are around plaques and they can be hit by "friendly fire" from the microglia, causing them to be damaged and maybe to form tangles.

It is not surprising that researchers have tried to link these two ideas: that mental activity strengthens connections between neurons and AD weakens these connections. To test whether there is a link, they first conducted epidemiological studies to see whether there is a correlation between one's educational achievement and the risk of developing AD. To do this, they examined a population of elderly people who would be old enough to have developed Late-onset AD. They ignored younger people whose risk of developing Early-onset AD would have been determined largely by genetics. Using medical records, the researchers separated the population into those that had AD and those that did not. Then in each group, they conducted interviews to determine each person's educational level. What they found is that individuals who did not make it past the 8th grade had a higher risk of developing AD, while those that completed four years of college had a lower risk of developing AD.

One possible interpretation of this study is that individuals with lower educational levels (either by choice, inclination, economics, or other variables beyond the control of the individual) are less likely to engage in routine complex mental activities putting them at greater risk for developing AD than those with college degrees. However, there are several limitations to these kinds of studies, which leave open several other interpretations. For one, there has been no conclusive study that has shown that individuals with different levels of educational achievement engage in different levels of mental activities during the course of their lives. Most of the experiments that have hinted at such connections have been done with lab animals where they have placed one group of rats in a large cage with lots of fun toys and compare their resultant brain structures to rats raised in isolation with no toys. From these studies, it seems pretty clear that the more enriched environment produced thicker cortex and more synapses. However, individuals who do not go on to a high school education are not living in an environment bereft of enriching stimuli, and thus extrapolating to the human condition is fairly tenuous.

Another possible limitation of the epidemiological study is that there might be another variable associated with educational attainment that causes one group to be more at risk for AD. For example, if one compares the income or net worth of a group of pre-high school dropouts to a group that graduated from college, one would expect to see a big difference. While wealth certainly does not prevent or lead to any physical disease, wealth can impact the type of medical care one receives throughout one's life. With consistent medical check-ups and access to more medical intervention, a person may receive more effective treatments for things like cardiovascular disease or infections. It is possible that such diseases might have secondary effects on the health and stress of the brain, which over one's lifetime can add up to enough physical damage to begin the pathologies of AD. If this is the case, then telling people to stimulate their brains to prevent AD is not the answer, but rather providing more consistent health care for individuals in all income brackets would be more effective in preventing dementia.

Finally, there is one more bias to consider for this type of study. The individuals who were diagnosed as having AD had this diagnosis based upon a medical exam. Unlike many other diseases, there currently is not a biological test to determine whether a living person has AD. Rather, a cognitive exam is given, where the physician asks the patient a series of questions to determine whether there is any dementia. In the case of Frank, his family was worried that he had AD two years prior to his eventual diagnosis. At that time, his wife took him to a physician who asked him questions like, "Name the last five American presidents in order." Frank, who read two newspapers a day and at least four non-fiction books a month, was able to answer the physician satisfactorily. There are plenty of individuals with no dementia who would have struggled answering such a question. Thus, it is possible that there is a diagnosis bias, creating more false positives in individuals with low educational attainment and more false negatives in individuals with high educational attainment.

With all of these limitations and other interpretations of the results, it may seem strange to even consider using these results to develop hypotheses and predictions. But these studies, warts and all, provide an excellent jumping off point to consider both what is going wrong inside the brains of AD patients and to consider ways of slowing or stopping the progression of the disease. Recent studies suggest that individuals over the age of 65 who engage in daily activities like reading books and newspapers and playing games like crossword puzzles and cards have more than a 40% reduced risk of developing AD. If the initial interpretation of the results is correct—that engaging in complex mental activities is correlated with less risk for developing AD—then there are at least three hypotheses which could explain these results: mental exercise protects neurons from the pathologies of AD, a well exercised brain is less likely to develop the pathologies of AD, or the potential to develop AD in later years decreases one's ability to succeed in education.

The first possibility is that one's educational attainment or how one "exercises" the brain does not affect development of plaques and tangles, the pathologies of AD. Rather plaques might form and tangles develop, but because there are more or stronger synapses, the unaffected neurons can still communicate effectively with each other and provide an effective substrate for cognition. The mechanism that is preventing an individual from developing the symptoms of dementia is the active engagement of neurons in complex mental activities which provides stimulation to create more synapses and/or strengthen existing ones. Under such a condition, an individual would be fated to develop the dementia that is associated with AD if that person lived long enough, but for a time, would be able to hold on to his or her mental faculties. While that might not seem like much, for the elderly it can be a great boon to know that there are a few more productive years to spend with spouse or to watch a grandchild grow.

Another possibility is that a stronger, well-exercised brain can resist more effectively the progression of AD pathologies. In section 2, we noted that scattered plaques and tangles may be found in the brains of elderly who are not demented. The problem in AD is not that these pathologies initially develop, but rather that they progress and spread and that the brain's ability to respond is not effective. Brain systems that are used frequently may be better prepared to deal with a physical insult that generates a few plaques and tangles, but prevents them from progressing further. One cellular mechanism that might be responsible for such a response is how a neuron deals with calcium. Calcium is a vital part of how neurons communicate with each other. Calcium is kept at low concentration inside of neurons while there is a high concentration of calcium in the spaces surrounding neurons. When one neuron communicates with another, pores open in the outer membrane of that neuron allowing an influx of calcium from outside of the neuron to the inside. The calcium inside of the neuron then activates a series of important chemical functions, including triggering the release of neurotransmitters, modifying the synapse, and contributing to electrical conduction within the neuron. Without this influx of calcium, neuronal communication would not be possible (Figure 10). However, there is a cost associated with this calcium influx. If the neuron does not get rid of the calcium quickly, it can build up to a high level and trigger a process whereby the neuron ends up destroying itself. In AD, some scientists have suggested that the presence of an A-beta plaque can disrupt the way a nearby neuron maintains a "safe" level of calcium. If degeneration due to the build-up of calcium occurs, the neuron could produce more A-beta or generate a tangle leading to the pathologies of AD. (Figure 11).

How would a well-exercised neuron withstand this progressive chain of events? A neuron that is constantly stimulated has more than likely built up internal structures to withstand large influxes of calcium. These cellular structures, called mitochondria and the endoplasmic reticulum, function to soak up excess calcium. By strengthening the connections in the brain via brain stimulation, one might be producing more mitochondria and larger endoplasmic reticulum. When a few scattered plaques develop in the brain of a person who has these more robust structures, the mitochondria and endoplasmic reticulum prevent the excess build-up of calcium preventing neuronal degeneration and the formation of more plaques and tangles.

A third possibility arises if one reverses the situation. Instead of considering whether high educational attainment and robust mental activities might protect against AD, it is possible that in some cases low educational attainment is due to an early, pre-clinical manifestation of

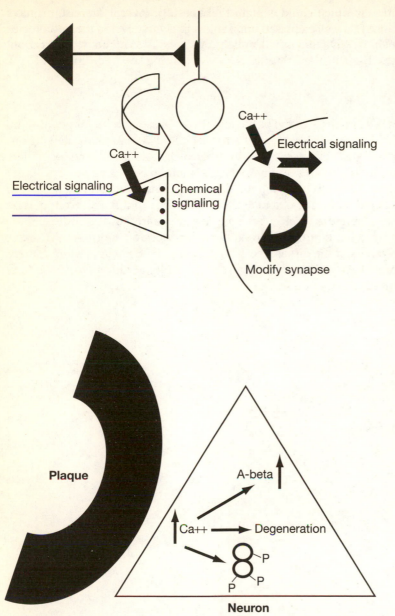

Figure 10
Top: One neuron (black triangle) extends an axon to communicate with another neuron (white circle) by making a synapse on one of its dendrites. **Bottom**: An expanded view of the synapse. Electrical signaling along the axon causes calcium Ca^{+2} to enter the nerve terminal which triggers the release of neurotransmitter across the synapse. These chemicals bind to receptors on the dendrite of the receiving neuron, and that can lead to Ca^{++} entering the dendrite. The influx of Ca^{++} contributes to the electrical signaling of that neuron so that it can communicate with its downstream targets. Ca^{++} is also used to modify the synapse to make it stronger and more efficient.

Figure 11
Plaques are thought to cause neurons to have a build-up of too much Ca^{++}. This unregulated increase of Ca^{++} may lead to the formation of tangles, the over-production of A-beta, and degeneration that could lead to the death of the neuron.

a biological mechanism that could lead to AD. A study that looked at a group of Catholic nuns that lived for decades in a similar environment, found that writing samples from when they were young were a good predictor of who developed AD when they were older. These writing samples were taken when they entered the order, decades before they were at risk for developing AD. The essays were analyzed and assigned a score of intellectual content based upon the vocabulary and syntax used. Those who ended up being diagnosed with AD had much lower scores on those early essays than those that did not have AD. One might argue that these results indicate that the nuns who developed AD in their later years did not have as effectively developed brain systems for processing language when they were younger as did the nuns who did not develop AD. This might indicate that some students who drop out of school are doing so because their brains are at risk for developing the pathologies of AD.

OTHER ENVIRONMENTAL INFLUENCES

Because there has been a dramatic increase in the past two decades in the number of people who have been diagnosed with AD, some have wondered whether there is something new in our environment which is contributing to this increase. A number of factors have been examined, such as whether the use of aluminum in our pots and pans is somehow poisoning us, or whether the electromagnetic waves that come from our appliances and power lines are killing our neurons. Scientists have conducted studies to examine these questions, and they have found no link between being exposed to aluminum or electromagnetic waves and the risk of developing AD. Most researchers have concluded that the most likely explanation for the rise in AD cases has been due to a greater awareness of the disease, both by patients and clinicians, which has led to more accurate diagnoses of AD. Also, with better health care and longer lifespans, the elderly population has grown, and will continue to do so.

Current and Future Strategies for Treating AD

As of early 2003, the Food and Drug Administration has only approved three drugs to specifically treat AD. All three of these drugs, Cognex, Aricept and Exelon, work in the same general fashion, by increasing the efficiency of communication across one class of synapses in the brain. These synapses use a neurotransmitter called acetylcholine to communicate from one neuron to the next. The acetylcholine synapses are just one of many different types of synapses that degenerate during AD; these synapses, however, are particularly important for storing and using memory in the brain. Each of the three drugs act by inhibiting an enzyme called acetylcholine esterase, which acts to break down the acetylcholine when it is released at the synapse. In a normal brain, the esterase is important because it limits the time that the neurotransmitter spends at the synapse, preventing the receiving neuron from getting too excited (Figure 12). In AD, with the acetylcholine synapses slowly dying away, blocking the esterase means that the neurotransmitter can stay at the surviving synapses longer, exciting the receiving neuron for a longer than normal time. By doing this, scientists believe that the diminishing number of acetylcholine synapses in AD could excite the neuronal networks similar to how a full complement of synapses could in a healthy brain.

This treatment strategy has only been effective for a subset of the AD patients, and then only for the first few months to up to the first two years that the patient has AD. During this time period, over half of the patients who take these drugs report some improvement in their daily living, their ability to think, and their memory. However, following the window of time when the medications are effective, patients suffer rapid loss in mental abilities to the point that they are at a similar symptomatic level as those who never received the medications. Researchers think that the drugs' effectiveness ends when one of two things happens, either so many of the acetylcholine synapses have degenerated that the surviving synapses are not producing a

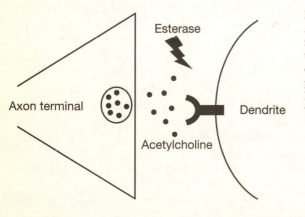

Figure 12
A cholinergic synapse. When a cholinergic axon terminal releases acetylcholine, this neurotransmitter moves across the synapse where it can bind to a receptor on the dendrite of the receiving neuron. An esterase (lightening bolt) is present in the synapse to break apart the acetylcholine, limiting the time the neurotransmitter can communicate with the target neuron.

noticeable impact on the neuronal networks, or other classes of synapses (ones that do not use acetylcholine) have degenerated to the point that it no longer matters whether the cholinergic synapses are being effective or not. The ultimate reason that the acetylcholine esterase inhibitors eventually fail patients is that these drugs are not designed to stop the progression of either plaques or tangles, nor are they designed to protect neurons from these pathologies. Not surprisingly, current research into designing future treatments for AD is focused on these two areas: combating the pathologies and trying to protect neurons.

PREVENTING OR REMOVING PLAQUES

As discussed in section 2, the easier of the two pathologies to consider blocking are plaques, since they form outside of the neurons whereas tangles form inside of neurons. Also, since the genetic data on the inherited forms of AD that we discussed in section 3 all point towards plaques as a more causative agent in AD, researchers have focused on these structures when looking for effective treatment strategies.

One of the most promising plaque prevention strategies has been the development of a vaccine that potentially might make one's immune system strong enough to block plaque formation. This strategy flies in the face of the study that suggests suppressing the immune system is effective in decreasing the risk of developing AD (section 4). When scientists gave an A-beta vaccine to mice that were genetically engineered to produce plaques, they found a huge reduction in the number of plaques that formed and the mice performed better on memory tests than mice that were not vaccinated. Animals given the vaccine did not show toxic side effects. Great enthusiasm was generated for the potential of this vaccine to fight AD. When a drug company began testing the A-beta vaccine in humans, however, there was severe inflammation, patients did not tolerate the vaccine, and they had to end the study early.

Researchers are trying to figure out why there was such a huge difference between the results of the animal and human studies. One possibility is that there might be crucial differences between the immune systems of animals compared to humans, and that a different type of vaccine needs to be generated to be effective in humans, especially elderly humans who are more at risk of developing AD and have weaker immune systems. Another possibility is that an AD patient's immune system is already active in trying to fight plaques and that the vaccine is unable to generate an effective response in the AD patient's brain. A third hypothesis is that the vaccine may have a different effectiveness depending upon the factors that ultimately lead to the generation of the plaques. In the animal model, the human genes for APP and PS-1, with the mutations that lead to early-onset AD, were engineered inside of them causing plaques to develop. In contrast, most of the humans who were in the vaccine study had late-onset AD without an APP or PS-1 mutation, and therefore the plaques were generated in their brains via different mechanisms and may not easily lend themselves to prevention by a vaccine. Finally, the vaccine may be effective in treating the early or even pre-clinical stages of AD, but be less effective and potentially even harmful at later stages in the disease. Because the pathologies of AD affect the immune system, generating a large activation of microglial cells, there may be a window of time when the vaccine approach could protect against the formation of plaques, but then lose its impact as the disease progresses.

Besides the vaccine approach, researchers are testing several other strategies to try to prevent the formation of plaques or to break them apart once they have formed. One is to find an enzyme that can cut apart A-beta once it has been released from cells so that it won't aggregate to form plaques. Another is to find a molecule that can break apart the A-beta after it forms into a plaque. Both of these strategies have had some success in experimental models and scientists are now trying to find effective ways to deliver these to the brain without creating a toxic reaction within the subject. Yet another strategy is to find a way to decrease the production of A-beta, thereby decreasing the likelihood or the rate of developing plaques. Two studies suggest that the sex hormones estrogen and testosterone could decrease the production of A-beta, while other studies are looking into ways to manipulate the secretases (proteins that cleave a molecule into different fragments) that cut APP into A-beta (Figure 6).

PROTECTING NEURONS

Another way to consider treating AD is to look at the health of neurons. If the progressive dementia of AD is due to the degeneration of neuronal networks, then finding ways to protect neurons in the face of the AD pathologies may be effective. Earlier we suggested that one possible way to protect neurons is to suppress the immune system because it might be damaging neurons around plaques. Two other strategies that are currently being tested with AD patients are the use of anti-oxidants and growth factors to protect neurons.

Growing old is the number one risk factor for developing AD, so it makes sense to consider fighting the effects of aging as a way of preventing AD. One current theory on the aging process is that as the body brings in oxygen and uses it to generate energy, molecules called free radicals are generated. If the body cannot eliminate these free radicals, they can destroy some of the chemical bonds that hold together and allow the proper functions of proteins, lipids and nucleic acids. As we age, our ability to get rid of these free radicals decreases, increasing the potential for damage to our cells. Neurons use a large percentage of the oxygen we consume, making them particularly vulnerable to free radicals. Some researchers have proposed that in AD, plaques increase the production of free radicals even more, contributing to degeneration of neurons in plaque infested areas.

Scientists are fortunate in that there are many known antioxidant agents that act as "free radical scavengers." Vitamins E and C, chemicals found in tomatoes (flavonoids) and carrots (carotenoids), and even the extract from the ginkgo tree (gingko biloba) are known free radical scavengers that are cheap and abundant in a number of foods and supplement sources. Several studies have shown that high doses of Vitamin E can slow down the progression of AD by 6 months in patients who are at the moderate stage of the disease (patients who are not yet institutionalized and can still feed and dress themselves, but who often fail to recognize long time friends or family members who are not living with them). With anti-oxidant treatment, these patients maintain daily living functions for an average of 6 months longer than those not receiving treatment. Current research is looking to see if Vitamin E can be preventative as well. Other studies are looking into other antioxidants like ginko biloba as potential neuronal protectors.

The study of early neuronal development suggests another way to protect neurons. In the 1940's a woman named Rita Levi-Montalcini discovered that a large percentage of the neurons created during an embryo's development die off during normal development. In some parts of the brain as many as half of the neurons die within the first few weeks of life. Over the next couple of decades, Levi-Montalcini and her colleagues found that neuronal survival is an active process, and that some neurons needed a chemical that humans produce called nerve growth factor (NGF) to survive. When more NGF was added more neurons survived; when the amount of NGF was decreased more neurons died. Recently scientists discovered that the mechanism of neuronal death that occurs in development might be similar to one of the mechanisms that lead to neuronal death in AD. That has led some to propose that finding ways to increase NGF production in the brain may protect neurons from the damage caused by AD pathologies. Unlike vitamins, large quantities of NGF must be produced in a laboratory, and even then there is no easy way to get it into the brain.

SUMMARY

The challenges for devising a successful strategy for treating AD are huge. Many scientists from all over the world are dedicating their research to gaining clues about the nature of AD and how best to combat it. In the years to come, we may find that the race to find a cure for AD will end like it did for Polio, with the development of a safe and relatively simple procedure that essentially eradicates AD from the general population. On the other hand, AD may more closely parallel cancer, a heterogeneous disease needing different strategies for management with a combination of genetic screening, recommendations for prevention (diet, mental exercises, vitamins, anti-inflammatory medications, etc.), and treatments designed to slow down the progression of dementia.

REFERENCES AND SUGGESTED READINGS

D. J. Selkoe. Alzheimer's Disease Is a Synaptic Failure. *Science* (298) 2002.

I. Dewachter and F. Van Leuven. Secretases as targets for the treatment of Alzheimer's disease: the prospects. *The Lancet Neurology* (1) 2002.

National Institute on Aging. Progress Report on Alzheimer's disease, taking the next steps. **http://www.alzheimers.org/pubs/prog00.htm 2000**.

S. Miranda et al. The role of oxidative stress in the toxicity induced by amyloid beta-peptide in Alzheimer's disease. *Progress in Neurobiology* (62) 2000.

R. B. Knowles, T. Gomez-Isla, and B. T. Hyman. A-Beta Associated Neuropil Changes: Correlation with Neuronal Loss and Dementia. *Journal of Neuropathology and Experimental Neurology* (57) 1998.

R. B. Knowles et al. Plaque-induced neurite abnormalities: Implications for disruption of neural networks in Alzheimer's disease. *Proceedings of the National Academy of Science* (96) 1999.

R. S. Wilson et al. Participation in cognitively stimulating activities and risk of incident Alzheimer's disease. *Journal of the American Medical Association* (287) 2002.

Y. Stern et al. Influence of education and occupation on the incidence of Alzheimer's disease. *Journal of the American Medical Association* (271) 1994.

W. A. Kukull et al. Dementia and Alzheimer disease incidence: a prospective cohort study. *Archives of Neurology* (59) 2002.

D. F. Swaab et al. Brain aging and Alzheimer's disease use it or lose it. *Progress in Brain Research* (138) 2002.

T. Tomiyama, E. H. Corder, and H. Mori. Molecular pathogenesis of apolipoprotein E-mediated amyloidosis in late-onset Alzheimer's disease. *Cell Molecular Life Science* (56) 1999.

S. Sinha and I. Lieberburg. Cellular mechanisms of beta-amyloid production and secretion. *Proceedings of the National Academy of Science* (96) 1999.

L. F. Lue and D. G. Walker. Modeling Alzheimer's disease immune therapy mechanisms: interactions of human postmortem microglia with antibody-opsonized amyloid beta peptide. *Journal of Neuroscience Research* (70) 2002.

J. Rogers et al. Microglia and inflammatory mechanisms in the clearance of amyloid beta peptide. *Glia* (40) 2002.

S. L. Chan, K. Furukawa, and M. P. Mattson. Presenilins and APP in neuritic and synaptic plasticity: implications for the pathogenesis of Alzheimer's disease. *Neuromolecular Medicine* (2) 2002.

M. Morishima-Kawashima, and Y. Ihara. Alzheimer's disease: beta-Amyloid protein and tau. *Journal of Neuroscience Research* (70) 2002.

D. Terwel, L. Dewachter, and F. Van Leuven. Axonal transport, tau protein, and neurodegeneration in Alzheimer's disease. *Neuromolecular Medicine* (2) 2002.

M. Sano et al. A controlled trial of selegiline, alpha-tocopherol, or both as treatment for Alzheimer's disease. The Alzheimer's Disease Cooperative Study. *New England Journal of Medicine* (336) 1997.

D.A. Evans et al. Prevalence of Alzheimer's Disease in a community population higher than previously reported. *Journal of the American Medical Association* (262) 1989.

L. Fratiglioni et al. Prevalence of Alzheimer's disease and other dementias in an elderly urban population. *Neurology* (41) 1991.